SRI JOYDIP ASHRAM

I0425391

INNOVATION@YOGAEDU-CATION

THE SRI JOYDIP ASHRAM STORY

SRI JOYDIP

9/22/2018

The ten years of Sri Joydip Ashram , had been a journey of innovation(reverse) on yoga education. Going out from the Swiss gymnastic model, which was popular 'one size fits all" yoga education methods, Sri Joydip Ashram in the last ten years, came with one after another, customised innovative methods on yoga education, which were both qualitative and safe, addressing the individual medical and psychological condition. The gripping story of Sri Joydip Ashram's ten years journey, of innovation in Yoga education; how it influenced beneficiaries, to come out in new ways of living with yoga, healing there medical and psychological condition would create value to every reader. At the same time the book gave objective and documented evidence in support of innovation in yoga education, in form of interviews of healing stories, where the beneficiaries shared their healing experiences.

1

CONTENTS

Appendices II : Some images of Yoga programs of Sri Joydip Ashram

Table of Figures

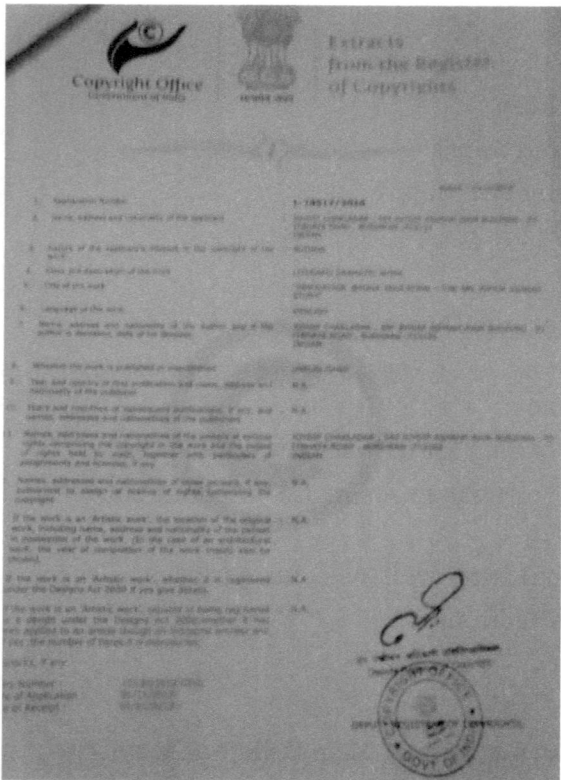

ACKNOWLEDGEMENT

In the tenth anniversary of Sri Joydip Ashram , the book is an humble effort, to present the Sri Joydip Ashram story, its innovation in yoga education. At the same time the author wants to thank on behalf of Sri Joydip Ashram, all the teachers , students, volunteers, well wishers , along with beneficiaries , who have helped us to reach us, where we are today.

DEDICATION

Yogeshwari – The Goddess of Yoga

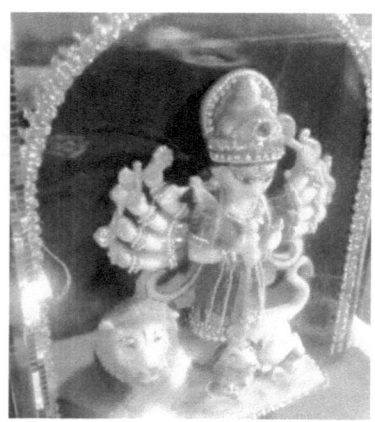

Three hundred million Bengalis, who are third largest ethnic community in world , waits for these four days, every year, in the remaining three sixty one days . A month long preparation goes to welcome her. Yet when she comes, only for four days, those days, becomes like four seconds.

Three hundred years ago, a man made a humble effort, to welcome her, in his palace. This welcoming still continues, in some different form, in a different place, for last sixteen years, by his descendants. Though there is no palace now, no huge arrangement, but the tradition continues with sincerity, devotion and creativity.

Every year Sri Joydip Ashram Trust, welcome humbly, the ten handed goddess, for last ten years , who is also known as "Yogeshwari" (one who is adept in Yoga) form of Durga, in her return jour-

ney, to her ancestral house, on behalf of
Sri Joydip Ashram community.

Why this Book and Why now ?

The top book on my category in Amazon, which is "Yoga and Meditation", is written by internationally acclaimed spiritual masters. At some point, it seemed to me a distant dream, that somebody will turn out, and go page by page, to read my work, in such a category.

So, I am earlier very convinced that people shall not read my work .

Why shall they ?.

I don't have gigantic ashrams, with millions of followers (though there is nothing wrong in having a gigantic ashram and a million followers) and great support from contemporary religious and political bodies. Last ten years, we have managed to remain, as far as we can, from some of the best opium for masses. Yes, we are possibly five hundred miles away, both from both politics and religion. The hindsight of it, is we don't pull as much crowd, as our work should pull, because most of the cases, crowd pulling happens not because of the merit of the work you do, but because how good and close you are, to this mass opium trends.

Whether they flied five hundred miles to come to us, or they just came walking five hundred metres, people who came to learn from us, came to us, because of the content of our thought, and not for our lifestyle. We live in very humble settings, with minimalistic comforts, and we believe our style of life, doesn't determine our quality of life. The quality of our life is determined, by the content, of what we think.

This is exactly what made me, rethink, about why people should read my work !

We don't have an ashram in the banks of Ganga, and we don't have it either around Himalayas, or in a religious town, where many spiritual stalwart stays. It can be easier for us, if we have our ashram on those environments. It is far more challenging for us, to have our ashram in surroundings, where culture of loud microphones , quarrels , thefts , violence are the order of the day . Still we have managed to stay as peaceful as we can, and heal people's mental and physical disorders from that zone, in the last ten years.

People and Organization, working for peace, can be disabled, and marginalised in many different ways, and Sri Joydip Ashram is one universal example of it. The culture of peace and compassion, which comes with spiritual practices like 'meditation and yoga', which is helpful to humanity, is always marginalised, because most people perceive it as a disability. In contrary, they perceive aggressiveness, violence and war, which are harmful, coming with politics and religion, as ability and cherish them in their ordinary lives.

From that context the stories, we tell about the bringing a culture of peace through innovations in yoga education, in the places, which are not known for them, becomes interesting; because of the frictions we have while travelling that difficult road. The stories also have a universal appeal that this understanding can be applied in other contexts too. We are not complaining, because everybody has their own share of friction, while travelling. We are just sharing our story, because we think, it could help many to face, that same challenges in a better way. They can also fulfill a lot of their spiritual needs of staying centered in difficult situation. Our resulting innovation on yoga education, to handle such difficult situation, people and things can also broaden the perspective of the reader.

Simply put , it is difficult to remain peaceful , as the incentive of peace is lower , and the incentive of aggressive and violence is higher . It is much more difficult, to remain peaceful, if you remain in environment of complete chaos and disorder. That's why story of Sri Joydip Ashram , promoting a culture of peace, by innovation in yoga education , in an environment of complete chaos and disorder is an interesting read for reader.So, the little success we have got in the path, needs to be also celebrated and shared with the reader.

Not always we are successful also, at certain things we have failed considerably. And we think that will even help reader on grasping, what we learned from them, as we have never stopped to make our effort, whatever the result, it may bring .

That's why I think it's the worth to read the book , and read it now, and leave a feedback and also encourage others to read it, and spread the word of mouth.

PREFACE

(Sri Joydip Ashram is a Public Charitable and Educational Trust , which operates under Indian Trust Law, 1882. According to Clause (6) of the Trust Deed the lawful purpose of the Trust is to disseminate Sri Joydip's Teachings , which are in the form of numerous Intellectual property like (Lifewise, Seven Yoga Habits that can Transform your Life , Creatiyoga, Workplace Wellness) which are created out of consciousness research in Yoga , for the benefit of the beneficiaries, who are the students of Sri Joydip Ashram, and also in Broader social context for public welfare.)

In this book, we are trying to both objectively and subjectively, find out how the intellectual properties of Sri Joydip Ashram are build, from its innovative education model, and how it is used further, to make a difference in the life of the Sri Joydip Ashram beneficiaries.

Some of the benefit programs, have evolved over a point of time in last ten years. Initially, these programs are named separately; then, these names evolved and became new names to be precise, on the benefits it brings.

At the starting point, there were more online programs, like 'Wisdom Stimulus benefit program', and 'Wisdom course benefit program', and then it was converted into new form of benefit program, according to the changing circumstances and nature of beneficiaries.

This are the list of benefit programs

Lifewise Benefit Program – Lifewise Benefit Program, is a unique yoga based life coaching program of (24 hrs and 12 days) spanned around 1 month, which teaches how to create "Work and Life Balance" and "Manage Stress" and "Live well" using Yogic principles.

Seven Yoga Habits Benefit Program – Seven Yoga Habits Benefit Program is a unique yoga based life coaching program of (100 hrs and 21 days), which teaches how to practice Seven Yoga Habits, for compassionate living.

Creatiyoga Benefit Program - Creatiyoga Benefit Program, is a unique yoga based life coaching program of (100 hrs and 21 days), which teaches how to improve creativity in life.

Workplace Wellness Program: How to be stress free and happy in Workplace is a unique yoga program for stress management in work, and improves the quality of work life.

Some of the foremost research question, we are trying to handle on the issue of innovative yoga education which Sri Joydip Ashram provides, in the
Sri Joydip Ashram story is following:

1. What is the innovation in the benefit program Sri Joydip Ashram brought in the Yoga Education, which has significantly improved the life of beneficiaries?
2. What are the principle thought, which guided this innovation, and who all benefited from it ?
3. What are the demographics, of these sample beneficiaries, and what are the kinds of changes they experienced, which can be told as complete transformation and beyond just body management.
4. What are social changes they experienced, when their bodies turned more sacred body with Yoga process?

Our idea is to also take a qualitative research approach, where we try to understand the Sri Joydip Ashram story, from both objective and subjective perspectives. So the book uses both narrative of an individual journey towards building one of the most innovative institution in yoga education, and at the same time, it also catches on the facts , figures and experience of the students, to give a more objective picture on the research questions.

What makes these book 'qualitative' is it offer ways to help us understand the complexities of Sri Joydip Ashram world, by exploring experiences of teachers and the students, and the supporting communities and the partners, the meanings they associate with Sri Joydip Ashram, the processes Sri Joydip Ashram follows , relationships it nurtured ,and the interactions it had, and also the social structures it was associated with.

THE SRI JOYDIP ASHRAM WORLD – DEMOGRAPHICS OF SAMPLE BENEFICIARIES AND THERE SHORT TERMS AND LONG TERM CHANGES

History of Sri Joydip Ashram

The Journey of Sri Joydip Ashram started with the virtual world and so it had a very dynamic virtual presence, and it students most of the time came from virtual world. The students also had the experienced the teachings virtually in the first two years of Sri Joydip Ashram existence .

However , from 2012 onwards Sri Joydip Ashram moved towards also making physical presence and presently from 2017 onwards the entire teaching is given physically, and online software's are used as supporting self-paced learning.

The principle hypothesis which was the context of building Sri Joydip Ashram is the
"inner creates outer" which is the experimentation that our inner thoughts , feelings and sensations, is creating the outer world be it virtual , or be it physical.

History of Sri Joydip Ashram in context of History of ancient civilization

In the two prominent ancient civilizations, India and Greece, which originated when human beings moved from Stone Age to bronze and Iron Age, we can see two distinct tendencies in the beginning of 3800 BCE. In Manjhadero and Harappa civilization, along with Vedic civilization, which came exactly after that, the same hypothesis, was dominant that it is only "inner which creates outer". We find the evidence of that from the archaeological traces of Manjhadero and Harrapa civilization and also from reading the literature of vedic times. The four vedas where we find the traces of the ancient socio-economic structures, we find the different deities, who are principles of nature and who are prayed for to maintain different aspect of the ancient civilization.

The satarudra, a part of Rig Veda, which was chanted regularly in Sri Joydip Ashram , is where Rudra , a fierce form of Shiva, is prayed for protection to maintain the different aspects of ancient civilization from cattle riding , to taking care of the family and at the same time to take care of wealth and well being. It was a time , when the early tribes are settling down into human habitats, after developing iron tools by which they are cutting forest, and so they are more close to nature then the present generation.

However, Greece took a very separate course and instead of observing their inner tendencies, they developed the early traces of scientific mind, trying to understand the outer nature and how to control it by tools and techniques, to develop the same purpose of protection of themselves and their community, along with wealth and well being.

When the Greeks attacked India , it was a clash of civilization and clash of principles. That was when the our forefathers of India, understood a need to develop a greater a political and social unity, and not remain divided into small units of Janapadas. This understanding is the basis of building the first Indian empire. The Mauryan empire was not build with a plan by the partnership of Chadragupta Maurya and Chankya the author of Arthasastra. It evolved around a need, a need to protect the Indian culture and Indian way of thinking from the Greek invasion. Vedic culture was not based on building empires, at the core it is liberal both in the thought and expression, and it is because of the force of external invasion, it had to build a force to protect itself and build the science of Dandaniti.

The formation of rigid organizational structure came out as a necessities when
Sri Joydip Ashram attracted international attention and there are students who started coming from different countries, who have separate culture then India, and who are very aggressive in nature, and who is primarily driven by externalities.

Building religion and building empire and nation, was never the primary intention of Vedic rishis. There primary intention was to make human being liberated from their mental conditioning and suffering, which they are subjected to.

This was also the intention of Sri Joydip Ashram, to build a small community of people where people educate and research to become liberated from the mental conditioning, they are subjected to using yoga as a tool and innovate education of yoga to meet the demands of present society.

However, when the Ashram continuously faced attack from the consumerist society which has invaded the para culture and nuclear family culture, where the outer socio economic status, starts ruling the inner spiritual culture, Sri Joydip Ashram, also has to come out from the sheath and start building an Organisation, where the inner work which we do for human well being is not exploited for political and social advantages and also everything was not decided on the base of socio-economic status quo.

As it is happened with the broader history of India , which come from the culture of peace , where war was pursued when it was absolutely necessary not just for to practise the game of war. A similar pattern also emerged in Sri Joydip Ashram , that we have to retaliate to protect our culture and hypothesis of "Inner creates outer" and our inner work and that's why we have to create a certain of Organisation to sustain our inner work and to restore our faith in Indian constitution. This is the foundation of Sri Joydip Ashram culture and work, and this is also the basis of our training programs.

History of Sri Joydip Ashram's work in Spiritual training

The Journey of Sri Joydip Ashram, started with the virtual world, and so it had a very dynamic virtual presence, and it students, most of the time, came from virtual world. The students mostly experienced the teachings on Sri Joydip Ashram, through different online tools in the first two years of Sri Joydip Ashram existence .

However, from 2012 onwards Sri Joydip Ashram, moved towards also making physical presence, where the teaching is delivered through instructor led classes, and from 2017 onwards, the entire teaching is given physically in a instructor based mode, and online software's are used as to support self-paced learning.

The principle hypothesis, which was the context of building Sri Joydip Ashram is the
"inner creates outer" which is the experimentation, that our inner thoughts , feelings and sensations, is creating the outer

world we live, be it virtual , or be it physical.

In each of the training program, we conducted, and designed we make it a purpose to keep working on this hypothesis, on exploring the inner world through yogic processes, and then taking this understanding and exploration to the outward world, to make significant changes, and feeding more data , that it can stand the fire of the critical review and scrutiny.

Sri Joydip Ashram platform, and the space , went through rigorous scrutiny, in these period of last ten years, sometimes by our teaching audit inside, and sometimes by the feedback we received, after the courses, and also while going through the courses.

In order to come up with the findings, and to stand on the test that the inner changes you make with Yogic process, can also make external changes in your personality and transform your body , vitality and your mind we also regularly published our finding in different yoga related publications.

Still the critical point remained, to be answer on the research question that "Do the idea of "inner is creating outer" is true for whole Sri Joydip Ashram community or its just limited to some individual cases ? ".

What is happening to the students, who have done the courses and have mild /medium/intense exposure to Sri Joydip Ashram education pedagogies?

What is the level of change they are experiencing after a short period of a month, a medium period of a year , a long period of ten years ?

The earliest student, of Sri Joydip Ashram. in the time of initial programs, is an South African lady (Kiki in 2009) right at the point of the starting of ashram, who got an intense exposure from Sri Joydip Ashram education methodology. However, though she gave positive feedback about the courses , there could not be any distinct changes documented ,as the training at that point of time was not so organised, and it was online through wiziq platform and very irregular .

The initial programs, are on different masters of Eastern traditions who have deeper connectivity with yoga philosophy like, Sun Tzu , Arthasastra and Sage Vyasa in Bhagvad Gita (one of the classic text of yoga) and also Shiva Sutras, delivered through online platform wiziq.

One of the earlier students, was also Hema Chocklingam and tamalian from United states, who maintained in touch with me still all these years, who first joined in the Shiva Sutras online program way back in 2010.

The training programs, when become regular from late 2010 with Bhagvad Gita courses running over a period of time , there was new group of students who joined .That is when, changes started with experience, of the students like Hema and Kiki and Rohit and Moumita , and slowly and gently they become more distinct .

There was also physical training program, on Bhagvad Gita which was joined Asit Baran Sarkar and he did the program for two long years from 2010-2012. At 2012 , we have also new group of students coming up like Ishita Sinha , Sha Sushmita Massi ,and we have students also from earlier Management background like Souvik Guha and Mainak Ball.

This students continued for next three years, with additional students joined in like Bhaskar Vaddavalli from US , Lida Cietro from Argentina , the students from Life of the Sage program, and students from different other institutions. The students have different level of problem from health to career, to concentration and mindfulness, and they wanted to address it through Yoga.

From 2016, onwards there was a new trend where students came very frequently with complex set of problems, and they wanted to get help from yoga on sorting them.

In the year 2017, there is an influx of International batches from different European countries, and also Indian families started incorporation the innovation of Sri Joydip Ashram Yoga education, for upgrading their lifestyle and incorporation the yoga for serenity and stress management.

The notable students here is Constantine Canon from Romania , Sutapa Ghosh from United States , Subhra Dutta from Denmark, and both the feedback of Subhra Dutta and Sutapa Ghosh after doing the program is recorded and there feedback is available online in youtube, and one can review those links and get a picture of there experience of the program .

The Feedback of Sutapa Ghosh (Psychologist from United States who is an Breast Cancer Survivor) after doing the 4 week long Lifewise Program, where 'Seven Yoga Habits for Transforming Life' is introduced to her, was, she had remarkable experience of pain management.

Living Seven Yoga Habits is a YouTube video which can be accessed on clicking the link and which documents the experience of Sutapa Ghosh, on going through the program.

Despite the influx of students from different cultural background and demographical set up, there has been a consistent success of the Sri Joydip Ashram yoga programs to give some short term benefit like relaxation, calmness, stress management happiness and also in long term, it healed some of the conditions of the students, both medical and psychological, related to different areas of life.

LONG TERM CHANGES – RECOVERING FROM ANXIETY ATTACKS AND BECOMING HAPPY

Still, there can be also a question regarding the events of outer change, and discourse of outer changes, and how it has happened with the programs, and what was the long term impact?

What is the language has been used to reflect and document this changes and how this is put together, to give an overall symmetrical picture ?

In 2019, we did a study on the long term impact of our program, where Subhra Dutta from Denmark, went through the Creatiyoga and Lifewise Program, and both the program have "Seven Yoga Habits" as a course material and she reported short term benefits with both of the program . She was suffering from problems with anxiety and having severe anxiety attacks and after doing yoga with Sri Joydip Ashram she was able to recover from those attacks both on short term and long term.

Rewinding 2018 with an Inspiring story is a YouTube video, which can be accessed on clicking the link and which documents the experience of Subhra Dutta, on the long term impact of the Sri Joydip Ashram program and how she handled pain and anxiety attacks gracefully and also build social relationships with more acceptance.

Hopes this serves as a good starting point of your journey to Sri Joydip Ashram World.

Welcome to Sri Joydip Ashram World where we represent the demographics of sample beneficiaries and there experience to give an objective understanding of Sri Joydip Ashram world. You can also find a new universe, which reflect the culture of peace and yoga innovation here , which can transform the reader in a very positive way.

NEUTRALITY OF
THE FINDINGS

I speculate that, there can be question that as Sri Joydip Ashram as an institution , which is founded by Sri Joydip , and being the writer of this book, have his own biases and prejudices, and probably not bringing the neutral viewpoint as it required to understand deeply, the innovation in yoga education, which was brought by Sri Joydip Ashram   .

However , my responded to this thought in this way

"However, when people came from different culture and background much of my cognitive biases and distortion on thinking, is removed from 2009 itself like Kiki from South Africa , Hema from US , Rohit from Lucknow , Sha Sushmita Massi from Malaysia and Ishita and Asit from Burdwan, and each of them brought more clarity. Further when we moved ahead, and have students from different countries things started self organising in itself as it happens with Yoga, that it has his own self organising energy which splits outside and create outer organization too."

So probably Sri Joydip's research and his work further, and many levels of testing is helping to make an organisation, which is perfectly defensible on next hundred years of its existence.

Then also the research has to bring, on exploring Sri Joydip's consciousness, and rigorously check that whether that consciousness itself is defensible that the outer expression of it, which is Sri Joydip Ashram also become defensible, in front of scrutiny.

RETRACTION

Sri Joydip Ashram , time to time received a lot of retraction, and scrutiny from peer communities, like other spiritual communities in Bengal and sometime other institute which questioned many aspect the poor infrastructure, we had earlier days, and also different the aspects of the teachings .

The question of retracting, due to recycling earlier work of research have also come , however , as it was explained that sometimes , this recycling is done to create a greater meaning and context of the present work, and explain the subtleties which was not included in earlier work .

Like the work Seven Yoga Habits that can transform your life , which is again referenced to find a deeper context , and turned into an ebook, like finding the root of "Seven Yoga Habits from Indian Gyan Yoga Literature".

However , in the last ten years one of my biggest realisation, is reliable and valid research is a powerful mechanism for change, innovation and problem solving be it in the inner domain of human existence or be it in the outer domain of human existence.

THE YOGA TEACHING TAPAS OF SRI JOYDIP ASHRAM

Teaching Yoga is a 'Tapas'. You have to do an intense practise in order to share the practise, that others could benefit from it. You have to practise your own practise for a longer period of time, that you can become master of it, and your positive flow of Yogic energy, doesn't get negated by the situation, people and things around you.

When I receive a call asking for a Yoga program, there are people mostly have many priorities, priorities about time, priorities about money. Surprisingly, the last priority seems to be, what they have made the call for – learning yoga.

Because, most of them have a wrong notion, that Yoga is very much the Swiss gymnastics and postural practise, which goes around it, and which has to be repeated everyday in similar way ignoring the holistic nature of yoga. (Montavon, 2014)

This 'one size fits all', kind of yoga, which requires routine drill, large footfall and viewership, are responsible for making yoga education taking a backseat and yoga noise front seat.

'You have to make a noise' the common social media principle has also invaded the yoga world in more negative ways, then in positive ways. Events have taken front seat, education is not even allowed backseat, certificate has become necessary, and learning is not even figured in necessities list.

The age old popular practise, whose intention is to relieve the suffering of human beings, is now engrossed in terminological wars.

What is important is not, how you name certain things, but how many people you can relieve from suffering, they are going through, both mentally and physically. That's how our fore-fathers the 'Rishis of India' , conceived yoga , to be a tool of inner technology , which relieves human being, from intense sufferings they are subjected to.

That requires innovation and creativity, and that's why yoga teaching is a tapas, where you have to continuously innovate to create aids, for alleviating suffering to help the beneficiaries.

As every person have different medical condition, physical con-ditions, emotional temperament and mental stability , the teach-ing has to be adapted , the learning has to flow according to the receptivity of the learner, the poses have to be adapted according to the personalities of the practitioner and there capabilities .

This is what, we are trying to do in Sri Joydip Ashram, with our limited resources in a humble way. It is not that the innovative benefit programs on Yoga teaching, in Sri Joydip Ashram, started with this book, or neither it will end with this .

Most of what we do in Sri Joydip Ashram , to help people/ beneficiaries alleviate there suffering, using yoga cannot be put in words , as Yoga is so intuitive, where teachers depends largely on his intuition, and the experience of his practise and teachings, to make the correct adjustments for his students to give him bene-fits of yoga, and to heal him from his medical and psycho-somatic conditions .

Yet this effort, is directed and aligned to the recent inclusion of yoga in academic circles, that the intuitions of yoga teachers,and his innovation and adjustments, for interest of the well being of the students, can be also documented and presented in a scientific manner .

THE VISION OF SRI JOYDIP ASHRAM

(This is the subjective experience of Sri Joydip while he conceived the idea of Sri Joydip Ashram)

In 18th Octobor , 2009 , I wrote in a small piece of paper "Sri Joydip Ashram" and I pasted that in my notice board . When I said, that there will be an ashram here people of my family , laughed at me . I was persistent to that idea, that there will be an ashram in the premises of my house, and nobody believed me.

In 2012 when I made a event , and also changed the structure of my premise, to make in an ashram, people started asking me can that be an ashram ?

Three years it went away make people believe, that I can create an ashram and teach spiritual lessons, and share my yoga lessons, even though I was teaching yoga for a decade, by then.

At 2012 , when I build the Sri Joydip Ashram trust, and try to make people join, they where many who are still was not trusting my intention and my work .

Automatically, I have crisis, failures one after another, yet the Sri Joydip Ashram could become a participant of United Nations Global compact , to gain trust of people , and also we did some excellent education programs like Wellness program , write a book called "Living Well" and at the same time do events like "World yoga festivals" where people started recognising our efforts on Yoga, and the peer community also started praising the work of

Sri Joydip Ashram.

The vision of Ashram , came as a flash of inspiration and intuition at the period of 2009 around 19th January , when I was meditating on Sri Aurobindo Ashram , Pondicherry . This was just an inspiration and there were no practical structures or support to turn this vision into reality.

It took seven years for me to articulate the vision, in a more clear terms at Decembor ,2015 when I decided to build an global Yoga Institution, which will work on the concept of human transformation, and human unity, from the stand point of "Vasudhaiva Kutubukam" which is a statement of Maha-upanishad, and a state of experience of how a person acts when he moves to the state of "Sthita prajna" of Bhagvad Gita which can be also told as "Brahma Stithi".

The state of this higher consciousness, can only take the manifestation, where the where one's concept of family is expanded to the entire humanity, and the selfishness and ego, has been transformed to one's higher consciousness. This is where one can work towards a higher unity of human beings through building Yoga habits, increasing their creativity, making their life wiser and workplace well.

With this vision Sri Joydip Ashram, started a new line of human potential development movement, through a deeper study and understanding of yoga, which can raise the human beings, to a higher standard of living.

Sri Joydip Ashram has the vision of building "Vasundhara campuses" which can house Sri Joydip Ashram, and also the Sri Joydip Ashram community , which can be like eco-cities all over the place energising transformation.

SRI JOYDIP ASHRAM'S MISSION AND IMPACT

Sri Joydip Ashram , is an institution, which delivers innovative education on 'Yoga' which has a tradition of ten thousand years , and the knowledge which was first delivered by the first Yoga Guru Sri Dakshinamurty to Saptarishis (The Seven Great Rishis) .

The Organisation and its system and process make an application of "Inside Out Model" of Yoga (Joydip, 2010) . According to the model, both inner growth in terms of meaning and spirituality, is sought with different yoga practices of excellence.

More importantly a balance, have been always sought between the inner and Outer growth. It is this balance between "Inner" and "Outer" makes Sri Joydip Ashram one of the most unique organisation across the world.

The Organisation fosters values of creating harmony between Individual growth and Collective growth, with the help of practice of highest form of Yoga , Spirituality and Transformational Management Practices .

Based on the "Inner Growth" it also practices the ideal of "Vasudhaiva Kutumbakum" which means to a person of higher consciousness, there is no stranger and everyone is a part of his family.

Vasudhaiva Kutumbakam (Sanskrit: वसुधैव कुटुम्बकम् vasudhaiva kuṭumbakam. From vasudhā", the earth; "ēva" = indeed is; and "kutumbakam", family;). Originally found in (Mahoupanishad) , the verse describes characteristics of a sadhak, who have reached the state of consciousness known as 'Brahma Sthiti'.

"अयं बन्धुरयं नेति गणना लघुचेतसाम् | उदारचरितानां तु वसुधैव कुटुम्बकम् || "
ayaṁ bandhurayaṁ nēti gaṇanā laghucētasām | udāracaritānām tu vasudhaiva kuṭumbakam ||

Discrimination saying "this one is a relative; this other one is a stranger" is for the mean-minded. For those who're known as magnanimous, the entire world constitutes but a family. (Mahoupanishad)

SRI JOYDIP ASHRAM'S OPERATING PHILOSOPHY

Sri Joydip Ashram's operating philosophy is imbibed with the principles of sustainable development, where not only financial but also social , and environmental bottom lines are taken care of, that a Organisation is created which could also secure resources for the future generation. Along with this lines , it collaborates with United Nations Global Compact, and participates in dissertation of 10 principles of Corporate Social Responsibility in Organization, across countries for making more inclusive organisation on Global Human Rights , Environment , Labour Laws and Anticorruption.

SRI JOYDIP ASHRAM EDUCATION PROGRAM

Sri Joydip Ashram which is legally an education trust, further delivers following short and long duration spiritual and leadership education programs, for realising its mission – a) Wisdom Programs b)Wisdom Stimulus c)Wisdom Program – Intermediate d) Wisdom Program – Advance e) Surya Yoga program for Health f) Wellness Program for Wealth and Wellbeing g) Guru Poornima Retreat – for advance and deeper spiritual experience h) Deepam Retreat – for advance and deeper spiritual experience. It also provides 2 research programs – 1) Advance Research Program on Vedic Philosophy and Management [2 years] , 2) Integrated Research Program on Vedic Philosophy and Management [5 years].

OXYTOCIN TAPAS

This programs often create experience of deeper faith, devotion, trust and forgiveness, and which also enables one to have a larger quantity of love hormones in their physical bodies which make there more loving, gentle ,compassionate .

There is an inner beauty which glows in the participants.

She has beautified her eyes with shades of black kajol. Though the drawing is discontinuous, At some places, still the voice and intonation, and way of throwing her speech can spellbound any hearer.

There is a form of joy thrives in her eyes and faces, which is captivating and yet when she get down from the bus , and walked towards her scooter , she was just like another simple women, covered her body with all encompassing shawl to encounter cold.

It was a chance interaction, yet it was touching deeply the memories, as the voice, act , and the whole movement has similarities with another women, who was an youth icon for him . The memories activated the brain, in a certain way and there is a release of a hormone which is called as oxytocin.

Popularly known as love hormone , this creates a certain feeling of wellness, in any human being who is experiencing the secretion of this hormone.

This hormone can flow not just by love , but also when somebody inspires the memory of what you love. Surprisingly , when you practice surya yoga , this hormone also secrets, and that's why practising yoga with Sri Joydip Ashram innovative yoga education in 'Lifewise program', also makes a person more loving and helps him to relate better the person near and dear to him , with the increasing secretion of oxytocin.

SRI JOYDIP ASHRAM STORY : BEFORE IT ALL BEGINNED

Did I planned to start a Ashram and innovate on the way Yoga education
is delivered ?
The answer would be big 'No'.

I had no plans to start an ashram or even teach yoga. I loved some practise of Yoga, and I shared it with people. Which later evolved, into benefit program, with significant number of beneficiaries? Initially, it was free and then after some time , we started taking some fees/donation for maintaining the expenses of running the program.

This is the way, all started way back in 2003, six years before I started the ashram operations, and then there was my involvement with other ashrams too. I was a regular visit of Sri Aurobindo Ashram. Initially , I was not interested on the philosophy and teaching of Sri Aurobindo . I just loved the place . I need some space to meditate, and it gave me some space. And after sometime , I became curious about what Sri Aurobindo is all about, and that is the time , when I elevated myself on becoming a student .

And then the relationship started .

16 years and counting ... my relationship with Sri Aurobindo Ashram continues,the yoga of savitri, and many unconventional yoga teachers, from ashram like Dr Jajati Bhattacharya , Arundhuti Di, Biswanath Da, Ananda Da , Larry , Alok Pandey, Shraddhavan , Shraddhalu the small study circle, where we continuously contemplate together, on the different aspects of the master work on Yoga , 'Sri Aurobindo's Savitri'.

In reality there was no plan , it just came spontaneously from my trekking to Himalayas, when I have my first spiritual experiences at the age of twenty years at 1995, sitting in front of Shivalinga mountains in Gharwal Himalayas and from there trekking around Arunachala a similar mountain without ice , fourteen years after in South India when I was age of thirty four.

In between I travelled the Kamakshya Hill , the mountains in Sikkim and WestBengal and also the ocean of Pondicherry , where I can manage to build a deeper and intimate relationship with nature.

And things took shape in it's own way of expression. So the culture of yoga practise took its own expression.

However , when went going deeper process and understanding, at some point of time , I felt my expression is getting stifled with the rigidity of some people, and that is where I need again another free space.

And this time , I have to make my own space, and that is how Sri Joydip Ashram came in shape . The space was so small, and it was intruded by some arrogant people , that I have no other way, but to opt to technology to give expression, of my new find interest, and also find more people with whom I can share my new love.

And this is how , I opted elearning tools, to deliver my education and teachings . My earlier failed effort on using online tools for educating people in 2007, this time became successful in 2009, when I started Sri Joydip Ashram , because I was really enjoying the freedom of expression, which I was getting and nobody is blocking my expression in any way.

That's how it all began . This was also a new time on the evolution of Bengal, where there is a lot of coming back to roots of Bengali culture then moving to an alien Marxist culture.

This shift was visible in Bengal's political landscape too.

That is how , we started teaching online in the banner of Sri Joydip Ashram from Octobor 2009 . We remember our first program was on "Art of War" . This classic of Sun Tzu, had always amazed me which includes deep thinking , detail planning and long preparation which is required for any wining.

Later , I started teaching Arthasastra , and then I was also amazed by the depth of the knowledge Kautilya possessed on statecraft , spirituality , war and almost everything, which was affecting the economic and social fibres of Indian society .

So, the back-story belonged to a series of conflict, which started from my home, and the jealousy between other house owners. The conflict did grow to my community, and also to the family, and at some point of time , it was also a part of my spiritual progress, and this is where, I need a space to experiment, with my own spiritual experience, and research my consciousness, and also to practise yoga and move ahead in my sadhana.

The existing structures are failing to give that support to me and I had to create something of my own, and that is how Sri Joydip Ashram got formed ten years back.

Reflecting on ten years of practise of Yoga, and teaching of Yoga in a framework of Sri Joydip ashram .

Stage 1 : Innovation with Wisdom Stimulus Story – 2009-2011

And then the tipping point happened , suddenly from January 2010, the backstory of my life, became the front story. I got an inspiration to share the teachings of Bhagvad Gita , with the idea of Wisdom Stimulus, when the world is going through Global Financial Crisis and the American Government, announced Financial stimulus to get over it.

I felt it was the lack of wisdom , and the corporate greed, which lead to financial crisis. And so at the same time , I also started an innovative online program, called Wisdom Stimulus, to give more in-depth idea, over the cycles of recession, which affect the humanity, and why did it come first place from a very yogic perspective.

It was instant hit to the online community, and people started joining the program from everywhere.

At end of 2010 , when a big Yoga teacher of International fame, visited the second tier town of West Bengal Burdwan, there was a lot of hype . There were two home grown yoga institution, they were very close to me. The rest of the institution are all, branches of the larger institution, which has main office , ashram or studios, in the capital of the state – Kolkata.

This is when the third home grown yoga institution Sri Joydip Ashram, came in place which from the time of birth, was coming up with innovative programs, and have a very global outlook.

Perhaps that is the reason today in 2018 , Sri Joydip Ashram's benefit programs of yoga, have many beneficiaries across the world, and some of them are leading institution around the world.

Some of the leading global institutes who are our beneficiaries

1.Diplomats and Library members of United States Consulate and American Library.

2.ETA Maelco (Dubai based International Organization)

3.NSIC (Government of India Organization)

4.Birla Corporation Limited.

5. Tollygunj Golfpark Residential Association

6. International Federation of Yoga Professionals

STAGE 2 : INNOVATION WITH YOGA HABITS , LIFEWISE ,WISDOM COURSE AND SURYA YOGA STORY – 2012-2018

At beginning of 2012, I also started teaching my first yoga program online , which is called as Learning Meditation Online . The program didn't work very well.

The biggest challenge any yoga program, faces is to design it to make it contextual the present living condition one is going through.

How can Yoga help to self organise, that one could handle the disruption of the external condition and the flux, which one goes facing on continuously ?.

This is the challenge of living yoga .

How do we bring yoga make those changes on life, which I know is essential for living well ?.

The failure of learning meditation online program, helped us to look at our yoga program design more deeply, and intensely and which make us think , that we have to considerably think, about the yoga habits, and also about the how body functions and how does it makes social influence.

And that's how ten years practise of Yoga, in different forms in Sri Joydip Ashram can be examined both from subjective and object-ive lenses.

When we looked from objective lenses, we can find the visceral experience of the yoga practitioner, once they have very domin-ant changes in their body in their movement, and in there inton-ation, which creates lot of new social interest.

And the most important innovation, came when Sri Joydip Ash-ram started observing the bodily functions and habits of a prac-titioner, and how they link to the social world, and how it trans-forms the social world altogether.

There are numerous observation of the participant facing num-ber of medical condition, what they understand Sri Joydip Ash-ram's yoga as a practise, internalise these practise and heals there condition with the help of Yoga.

This experience of them , is recorded on the forms of videos and statement, from numerous participants who are beneficiaries of the programs.

There are both Short term benefits, and also long terms benefits, which people gained from Sri Joydip Ashram Programs

Some of the students experience and for some we have their statements in pictures and we have listed them here just to give an idea of what is the kind of experience Sri Joydip Ashram Pro-gram Creates.

1. Ishita Sinha (2012) – Burdwan- Experience of Wellness Program

2. Tapas Rui Das (2015) - Burdwan -Experience of Wellness Program
3. Leda Cecilo Citro, Certified Yoga Teacher ,
   Yoga Alliance ,Argentina (2014) – Argentina – Experience of Wellness Program
4. Sutapa Ghosh (2017) – USA – Experience of Lifewise Program
5. Subhra Dutta (2017) – Denmark – Experience of Creatiyoga Program
6. Kalyani Chatterjee (2017) – Kolkata – Experience of Lifewise Program
7. Amitava Ghosh (2017) – Burdwan – Experience of Lifewise Program
8. Manish Verma (2018) – Bangalore – Experience of Lifewise Program
9. Nandini Biswas (2018) – Burdwan – Experience of Lifewise Program
10. Srinivas and Jyoti Pasumurti (2018) – Experience of Lifewise Couples Program

This ten students which are a sample of students, from ten years of time , reflect their experience on how Sri Joydip Ashram's yoga programs, support the cognitive , development and creates happiness and peace, and positive yoga experience for cross sections of learners.

The teachings of Sri Joydip Ashram, was made through sharing the being on demonstration the divine experience of peace , bliss and happiness. The core of teaching is gravitated around application of Yoga in life conditions (lifewise , building yoga habits , inspiring creativity , and managing stress in workplace) and the learning experience involved doing things, that change one's objective and internal environment . This particular set of teachings, is also emphasised in one of sub schools of the six school of Indian philosophical thoughts which is known as "dristi-sristhi advaita", "whatever you see , that is what it becomes".

Though the observation was initially gravitated around the body management but slowly and gently when the participant deepened, there practise they often realise how much of emotional , spiritual transformation, which they started experiencing just between three months of starting of the yoga workshops with Sri Joydip Ashram.

Most of the Sri Joydip Ashram benefit programs, are started from week long program to three to six months long . However from the late 2016, the programs started ranging from one week to seven week , between three days to forty eight days and between ten hours to five hundred hours . A list of programs which have been conducted both online and offline, under the banner of Sri Joydip Ashram is given here

1. Art of War (2009)
2. Arthasastra (2009)
3. Wisdom Stimulus (2010-2012)
4. Shiva Sutras (2010-2017)
5. Learning Meditation Online (2010)
6. Wisdom Program (2012)
7. Guru Poornima Retreat (2012-2018)
8. Deepam Retreat (2012-2016)
9. Bhakti Yoga Courses (2013)
10. Wellness Program (2014)
11. Surya Yoga Program (2014)
12. Lifewise Program (2018) – Copyrighted
13. Seven yoga habits (2018) - Copyrighted
14. Creatiyoga (2018) - Copyrighted
15. Workplace Wellness (2018) - Copyrighted

Near about twelve programs is executed, in the period of ten years to different age groups both online and offline and they focus on following areas

1.Yoga Philosophy

2. Postural sequence and Breathing exercises

3. Anatomy and Philosophy

4. Understanding physical and energetic body

5. Meditation

6. General Fitness

7. Healing Disease

8. Yogic Diet and how food could be a medicine

9. Workplace Wellness

Mode of education in this yoga program are

1. Self study through online program Sri Joydip Ashram online Yoga Varsity
2. Instructors Training
3. Teachers Training
4. Continuing education opportunities

The continuous innovation of Sri Joydip Ashram program designing team, helped to take the feedback of the students, and design new learning experiences, for specific age groups help to design, implement and facilitate learning experiences.

1. Kids
2. Young Adults or Teens
3. Adults
4. Medium Aged
5. Old Age

There are evidence that Innovative Yoga intervention of Sri Joydip Ashram in form of different programs, helped to relieve mental health and physical health consequences.

There are yoga based whatsapp and knowledge communities, which are build to enhance the learning experiences, in different programs. This entire benefit programs with yoga intervention, where different people continued, over a period of time, and the programs are used as a tool for people suffering in different physical and mental conditions to explore their inner landscape.

Many participant who are unable to choose a life, outside the trapping of her circumstance , Sri Joydip Ashram innovative yoga education benefit program, gave a hope to those beneficiaries, that adopting yoga practise, that resonates with her , they can, she will able to carve out space, within the circumstance ..

Reverse Innovation with Yoga : Sri Joydip Ashram approach

One of the areas, where Sri Joydip Ashram benefit program, was trying to improve on the social power of beneficiaries , specially people, who are patient who are suffering from mental disorder, and problems in social communication. The bodily knowledge and awareness which is grown by yoga, helped them to improve social skills to the beneficiaries. While going through this benefit programs, many participant, which had lack of social potential, and they could connect the society in a very different way.

While giving the yoga teachers training , Sri Joydip Ashram first put the apprenticeship process in practise , where teachers not only observe the process , when they demonstrate , but they feel the process, and there is certain degree of visceral experience which comes towards him , which transform them spiritually , emotionally and psychologically.

Yoga is already as a reverse innovation tool, an innovation which is moving from an developing country to an developed country.

On that way , Sri Joydip Ashram was driving its innovative yoga teaching, with a group of volunteers , using the power of Internet, and reaching out people across the world ten years back when the technology in India, on terms of Internet is still evolving is definitely an innovation.

On the top of it building customised modules , moving away from lecture based and Swedish gymnastic and traditional military drill based training, how yoga classes where taught in west, is surely an example of reverse innovation where the adaptation is coming slowly and gently.

The real innovation, was on the model too, where we started from assessment and then moved to the sequence, where there was a lot of scope of customisation of the sequence, and then there was a scope of alignment towards the sequence and moving towards a home practise, with an set way of doing things in a very customized way, is definitely and innovation in yoga education.

SRI JOYDIP ASHRAM TEACHERS TRAINING

At 2017 , Sri Joydip Ashram also felt a need to build innovative yoga teachers, and extend their beneficiaries across the world, and the ashram started taking application for teachers training across the world.

There are participants, who applied for teachers training in Sri Joydip Ashram,on following beneficiary program format

1.Lifewise Yoga Teachers Training (Residential)- 7 weeks / 48 days / 500 hrs residential program

2. Lifewise Yoga Teachers Training (Non - Residential)
7 weeks / 48 days / 100 hrs non residential program

The Ashram received applications from following countries

1. Israel (2)
2. Romania (1)

3. France (1)
4. Sweden (1)
5. America (3)
6. Estonia (1)
7. India (1)

There are two students from Romania and Estonia in Europe, who can completed the requirements of the Sri Joydip Ashram Yoga Teachers Training program . They are Constantine Canon-(Romania) and Anti Kesama (Estonia) and got the rights to teach Sri Joydip Ashram programs in Europe.

However it is the first time , we also faced a different kind of thought turmoil, on Yoga mostly coming from western origin . The yoga lifestyle, there has a consumptive quality, which also brings some good things, like cultural atmosphere of reinvention, merging with profit and personal purpose. There is also a moving nature of yoga in western landscape in Europe and America, where its is a "centre of creativity" . It is entrepreneurial, business oriented, branded and marketed for consumption.

With this International students , Sri Joydip Ashram also has innovate further to balance with the learning requirement of students. For this we have to move through transdisciplinary enquires which involve studying psychology , sociology , intercultural studies .

There is also one student who came lately from India, Kumari Pratiksha, who completed the 7 weeks / 48 days / 100 hrs non residential program in Yoga from India . And she became the first Lifewise Yoga Teachers from India (Kolkata).

The Yoga Teachers Training, also used many innovative methodology of training the teachers and one of them is "Live Yoga Teaching" in Lifewise Yoga Teachers Training, which was for non residential yoga teachers training program.

In the residential the participants are asked to participate in Yoga conference like "Green Yoga" and "Gyan Yoga Tradition" , and selecting a research topic in Yoga and trying to build innovative research oriented papers in Yoga, and presenting them in the conference.

There is a huge difference between Sri Joydip Ashram approach to yoga, for curing disease to the medical approach to disease. The medical approach or the biologist approach is reductionist, where every living organism is turned into chemical substance, and the only ways seems to heal the disorder to reorganise that chemical substance in every possible means. Whereas Sri Joydip Ashram approach towards yoga, is more holistic, where not only physical body is taken care, of but associated pranic body and other layers of mental and intellectual body known as manomaya and vijananmaya kosha is also taken care of.

CONCLUSION

Honestly , there is no conclusion of the building of the adaptation of the teaching philosophies and practices of Yoga, which are continuously experimented and innovated to meet the demands of different beneficiaries coming from different countries who want to use Yoga for different causes.

Sri Joydip Ashram, continues to evolve with the set of challenges it faces, on day to day , basis to address the different problems, on different age groups through Yoga. However , we also want to mention that Sri Joydip Ashram innovation in Yoga education, is less academic , where people are spending years and years, on doing different aspects of research in Yoga, and they have adequate funding for that purpose. We find our research and innovation is more agile and applied, and there is a continuous loop of feedback, we went on receiving from our students and beneficiaries, and which helped us to adapt and correct ourselves.

Besides, we don't have such resources till now, and we had to do the research mostly from our internal funding mechanism, and most of the time , still the beneficiaries get a lot of results, because of the innovation, we have done through Yoga.

Probably we felt in the process , if we had documented it better , then obviously there are more beneficiaries, who could have benefitted from our effort on bring innovation in yoga education, which are both safe and also had a very high quality.

This book, is a attempt on that direction where our reader can learn about our innovation in yoga education and benefit form them. We could also reach out more people who are in the dire need of new ways to solve their old problems through Yoga.

BIBLIOGRAPHY

Joydip, S. (2010). *The Integral Management - Principles and Practices.* Kolkata: Lulu.

Montavon, A. A. (2014). *YOGA TEACHER TRAINING CURRICULUM DESIGN:.* United States: UMI.

APPENDICES I :
SHARING SRI JOYDIP
ASHRAM MAIN
BUILDING STORY

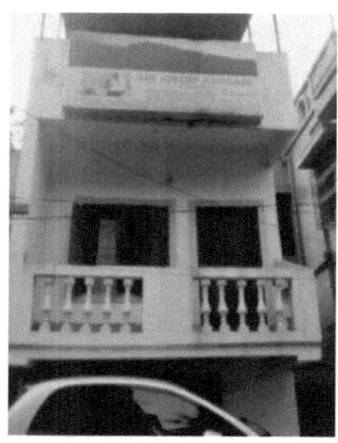

Build on Year 2003 , the earlier the building was used as a Meditation Hall for teaching Reiki , yoga and different other spiritual practices . However , after the ashram was formed the building was also housing the students of the ashram and giving them training . In 2012 , when the trust deed was developed , the entire building went through structural changes, and presently the whole building is used for Sri Joydip Ashram operation and is known as Sri Joydip Ashram main building.

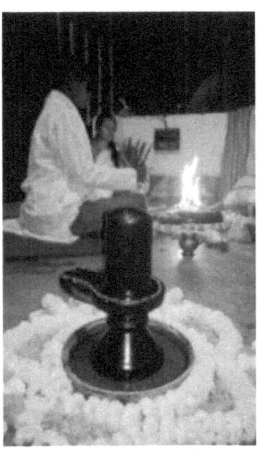

Appendices II : Some images of Yoga programs of Sri Joydip Ashram

FIGURE 1 : SRI JOYDIP ASHRAM YOGA PROGRAMS IN US CONSULATE

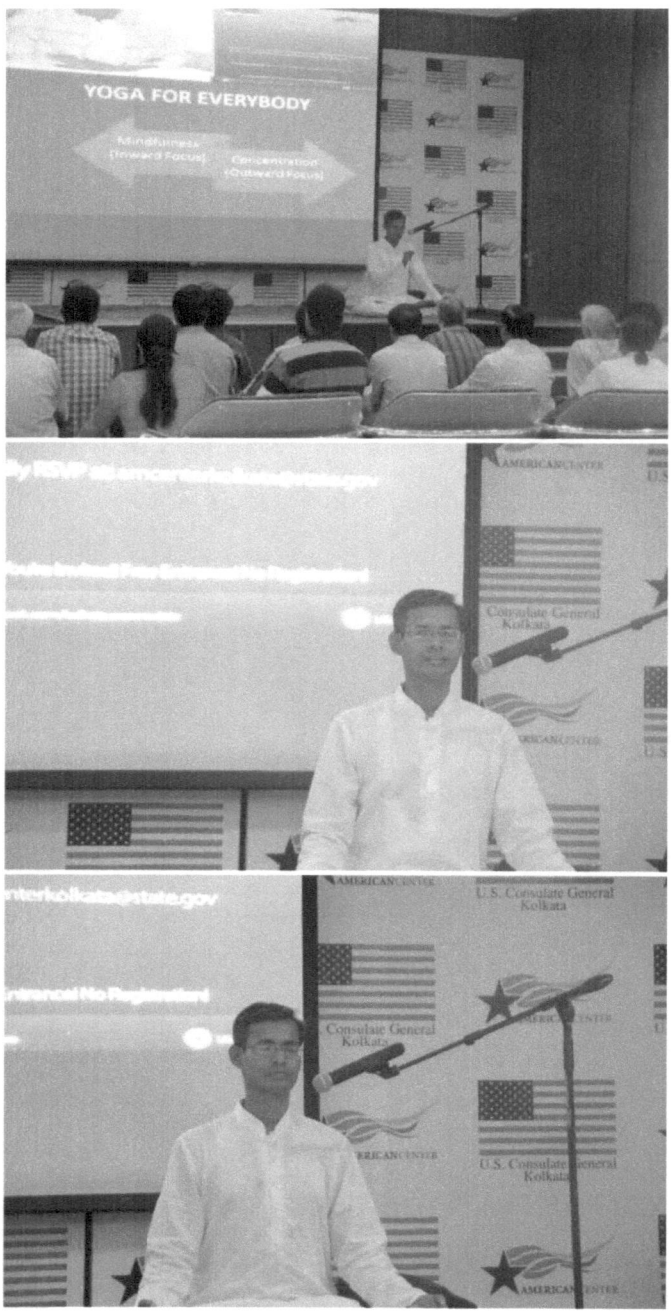

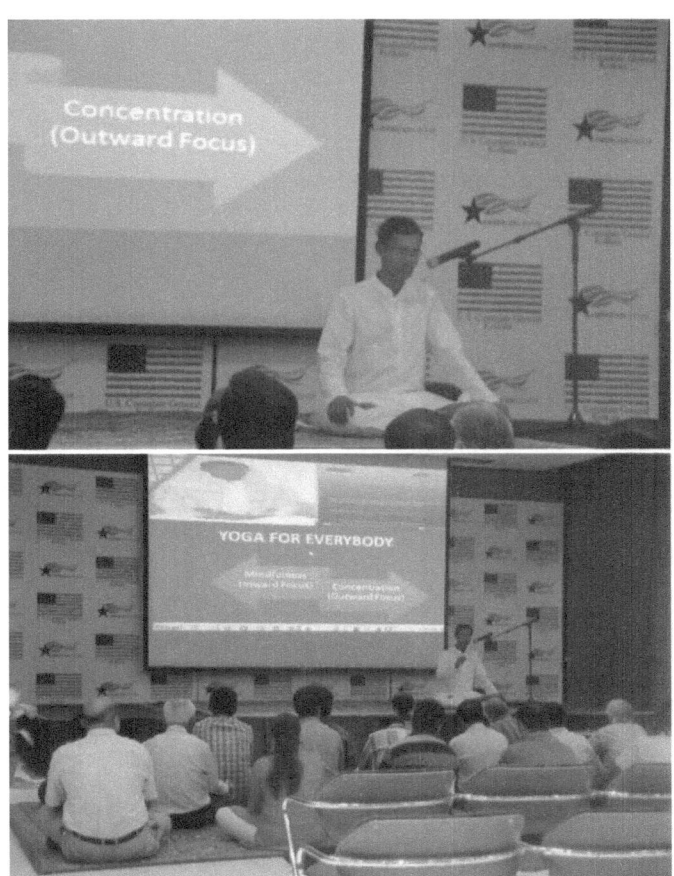

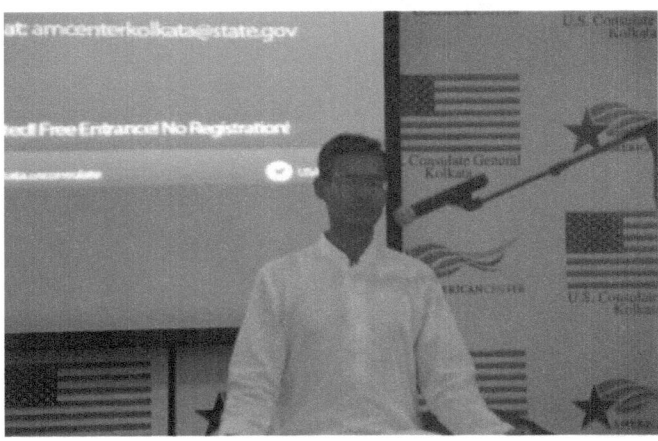

FIGURE 2 : SRI JOYDIP ASHRAM YOGA PROGRAMS IN DIFFERENT PLACES

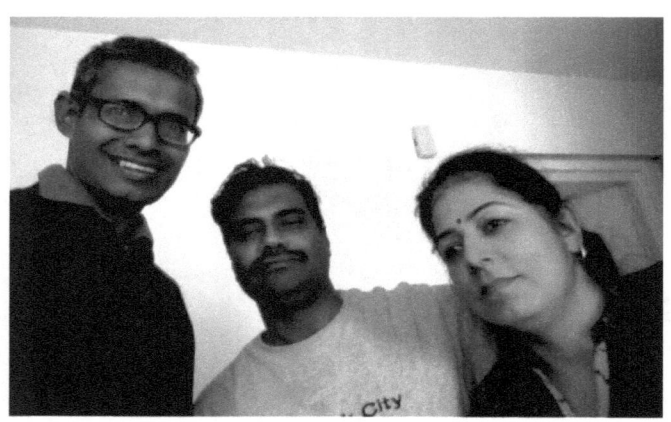

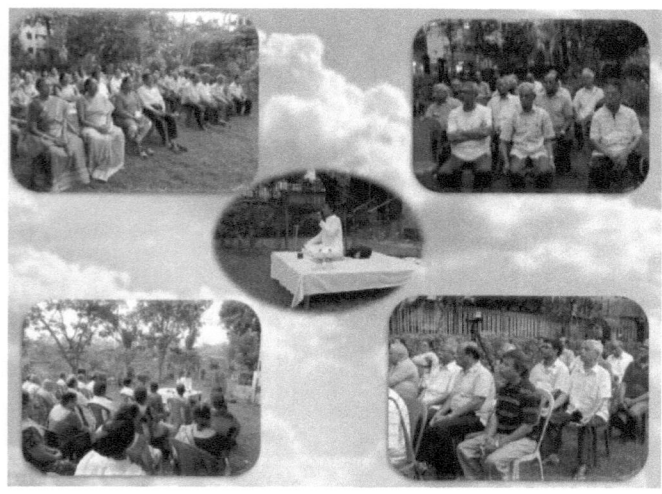